DIABETIC DESSERT COOKBOOK

Diabetic and Prediabetic Guilt Free Guide to Prepare Delicious Low carb and Low Sugar Desserts, Cookies, Bread and Cakes that Whole Family Can Enjoy for Healthy Sweet Moments

Oliver Hendry

brands within this book are for clarifying purposes only and are the owned by the owners themselves, not affiliated with this document.

Table of contents

Introduction

Maintaining a healthy weight is vital for everyone, but if you have diabetes, excess weight can make your blood sugar levels more difficult to control and may increase your risk of some complications. Weight loss can be an extra challenge for people with diabetes. You need to eat healthily as you seek to lose weight, but if you have diabetes, eating the wrong diet may harm your health. Pills for weight loss and diets for malnutrition can be avoided at every cost but several common diets can be helpful.

You must focus on consuming lean protein, fewer carbs, and no processed food, high-fiber, fruits and vegetables, dairy with low fat, or if you can find it fat-free, and healthy vegetable fats such as nuts, avocado, olive oil or canola oil if you have diabetes. Your food consumption will be handled as well. Having your doctor or dietitian have meals and snacks with a specific carb level. In total, women should be aiming about 45 grams of carb per meal and men should be aiming 60. It will preferably come from dynamic grains, nuts, and vegetables.

The American Diabetes Association offers a detailed guide regarding the best foods for people with diabetes. The recommendations include:

Proteins: beans, eggs, poultry, nuts, and salmon, sardines, and tuna.

Dairy: non-fat or low-fat yogurt and non-fat or low-fat yogurt.

Fruits/Vegetables: sweet potatoes, berries, and okra, kale, asparagus, and broccoli.

Grains such as whole wheat pasta, whole grains; brown rice.

Staying hydrated is critical in terms of physical safety, too. Whenever necessary choose non-caloric alternatives such as water and tea.

Chapter 1. Kinds of Diets Good for Prediabetic or Diabetic Persons

Certain foods should be limited to people with diabetes. These foods may trigger blood sugar spikes or contain harmful fats.

They cover:

- Grains cooked, for example, white rice or white pasta

- Introduced sweetening foods, including apple sauce, jelly, and some canned foods

- Full-fat dairy

- Products fried or heavy in trans fats or saturated fats

- Products produced from fine wheat

- Every product that has a heavy glycemic value

1. The dietary approach to stop hypertension (DASH) plan

Originally intended to better manage or avoid high blood pressure (hypertension), the DASH program may also decrease the likelihood of certain diseases, also diabetes. This will even have the additional advantage of helping you drop weight. People who follow the DASH diet are encouraged to reduce portion sizes and eat foods rich in nutrients that lower blood pressure, such as potassium, magnesium, and calcium.

The DASH meal program contains:

- Protein lean: Fish, Poultry

- Foods based on plants: vegetables, fruits, beans, nuts, seeds

- Dairy items: animal goods free of fat or reduced in fat

- Whole grains

- Healthy fats: Oils from vegetables

In this program, it is advised that people with diabetes limit their sodium consumption to 1,500 milligrams a day. The program even bans chocolate, sugary drinks, and red meats.

2. The Mediterranean diet

This diet is influenced by typical Mediterranean diets. This diet is rich in oleic acid, a fatty acid naturally present in fats and oils based on animals and vegetables. Countries known to eat from this diet include Greece, Italy, and Morocco.

According to research in Diabetes Spectrum, a Mediterranean-type diet may be effective in reducing glucose levels, lowering body weight, and lowering the risk of metabolic disorder.

Foods eaten during this diet shall include:

• Protein: salmon, poultry, fried fish and other species

• Food dependent on plants: fruit, vegetables such as artichokes and cucumbers, beans, nuts, seeds

• Good fats: coconut oil, almond nuts,

Red meat can be eaten once a month. Alcohol should be drunk in moderation because it can improve cardiac safety. Remember you should never drink when you have an empty stomach if you are on medicines that increase insulin levels in your body.

3. The Paleolithic Diet

This diet focuses on the assumption that the responsibility for chronic disease rests with modern agriculture. Paleo diet adherents consume only that which our ancient ancestors may have hunted and harvested.

Foods consumed during the Paleo diet include:

• Protein: meat, fish, poultry,

- Non-starchy foods: grains, fruits, seeds, nuts (excluding peanuts)

- Balanced fats: walnut oil, avocado oil, olive oil, coconut oil, flaxseed oil

A paleo diet is a good option for persons with diabetes as long as the person has fine and healthy kidneys. A paleo diet can boost glycemic regulation in the short term for people with type 2 diabetes, according to a three-month analysis reported in the Journal of Diabetes Science and Technology.

4. Vegan or Vegetarian Diets

Any diabetes sufferers focus on consuming a vegetarian diet. Vegetarian diets usually apply to diets where no meat is consumed, but may contain animal items such as milk, poultry, or butter. Vegan individuals do not consume beef or other food items, including honey, butter, or gelatin.

Foods that are healthy for vegetarians and vegans with diabetes include:

- Soy

- Fruits

- Beans

- Leafy vegetables

- Legumes

- Nuts

- Whole grains

Although vegan or vegetarian diets can be healthier diets to adopt, if not vigilant, those that pursue them might be losing out on crucial nutrients.

Some nutrients vegans or vegetarians might need to consume using supplements include:

- Iodine. The iodine required to metabolize food into energy is contained primarily

- in seafood. Without these animal items, vegetarians or vegans may have difficulty having enough of the requisite iodine in their diets. Supplements, however, can help.

- Zinc: The primary supply of zinc is from high protein meat foods, so anyone with a vegetarian diet will be recommended to provide a replacement.

- Calcium. Calcium found mainly in animal products such as dairy, is an essential nutrient that contributes greatly to bone and teeth health. Kale or broccoli may help provide the calcium required, although a vegan diet may require supplements.

- B-12: Because only animal products have vitamin B-12, anyone adopting a strict vegetarian diet will need to use a supplement.

5. Gluten-free diet

Gluten-free diets have been common but the removal of gluten from the diet is important for people with celiac disease to prevent harm to the colon and body. Celiac disease is an autoimmune disorder that triggers an attack on your gut and nervous system by your immune system. It also causes inflammation in the body and may contribute to chronic disease.

Gluten is a nutrient present in maize, rye, barley, and other grain products. 10 percent of people with type 1 diabetes often have celiac disease, according to the American Diabetes Association.

Tell the doctor to perform a celiac disorder blood check. You may also be intolerant of gluten even though it falls low. Talk to your doctor about whether you should have a gluten-free diet.

While anyone with diabetes may take a gluten-free diet, it may introduce restrictions for anyone without the celiac disease. Recalling that gluten-free is not equated with low carb, too. Processed, high-sugar products that are gluten-free are available. There's usually no such need to make meal planning complicated by eradicating gluten until you need it.

Physical activity is important for the wellbeing of people with diabetes in addition to having the correct diet. Exercise can help to reduce rates of blood sugar and A1C and may help to prevent risks.

Even if you see improvement with physical exercise, don't change your prescribed insulin routine without your doctor's advice. If you are taking insulin and trying to add or implementing adjustments to your fitness routine, test before, during, and after exercise. This is true even if you think the weight gain is caused by the insulin. Changing your insulin schedule could affect your blood sugar levels. These modifications may trigger problems that could endanger life.

If you're worried about your weight, speak to a doctor or nutritionist. They will help you choose the lifestyle that fits your unique dietary requirements and expectations for weight loss. They can also help avoid food and drug problems and can interfere with prescription drugs.

Chapter 2. Recipes for Low-Carb and Low-Sugar Desserts, Cookies, Cakes, Bread and More

A healthy diabetic diet is all about equilibrium. As long as moderation is taken into account, the total amount of carbohydrates in your diet makes up a small amount of sugar. As a general rule, diabetics will seek to cut down on products and beverages that contain high levels of sugar as they can find it more difficult to regulate blood sugar and weight. If you adopt a diabetic diet, these smaller, safer treats are good sweets to think. All of these 45 dishes are around 30 g or fewer carbs per meal.

1. Cream Cheese Brownies

It takes 20 minutes for preparation and 25 minutes for baking. You can make 1 dozen brownies with the following ingredients.

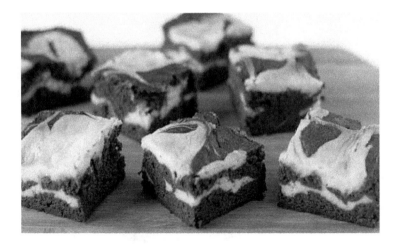

- Large eggs (3)

- Soft, low-fat Butter (6 tablespoons)

- Sugar; 1 cup

- Half cup flour (all-purpose)

- Baking cocoa; ¼ cup

- Low-fat cream cheese; 8 oz. 1 Packet

Preheat the oven to 350 ° C. Set aside 2 eggs separately, place each white in a bowl (save for later use). Beat butter and 3/4 cup sugar in a small bowl, until crumbly. Beat 1 egg white and vanilla in the remaining whole egg until well combined. Combine the flour and cocoa; slowly transfer until combined to the egg mixture. Pour into a 9 inches square pan for baking. Line the pan with cooking spray; set away.

Beat the remaining sugar and the cream cheese in a bowl, until smooth. Beat white in the second shell. Fall into the batter by rounded tablespoonfuls; slash into the batter to churn with a knife.

Bake for 25 to 30 minutes or until complete, then take the edges from the sides of the plate. Cool it down on a rack of string.

2. Tiramisu Cake

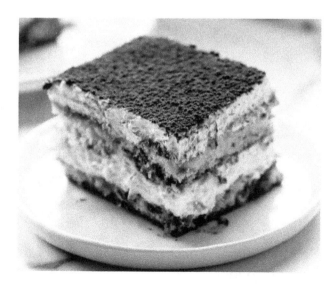

This cake requires 25-30 minutes for preparation. You can easily prepare 9 servings with these ingredients.

- Baking cocoa

- Ladyfinger cookies (24)

- Heavy cream; Half cup

- Vanilla yogurt; 2 cups

- Fat-free or low-fat milk; 1 cup

- Strong coffee or espresso; Half cup

- Raspberries (optional)

Beat the cream in a small bowl until it gets stiff; fold yogurt. Place 1/2 cup cream mixture over an 8 inches dish.

Mix the milk and espresso into a shallow dish. Dip 12 ladyfingers into the coffee mixture quickly, allowing excess drip away. Set in a single layer in the dish, breaking to fit as required. Fill with half the remaining milk mixture; cocoa wax. Repeat across walls.

Cap, refrigerate, at least 2 hours before eating. Serve with raspberries if you prefer.

3. Ginger Plum Tart

This tart requires a total of 35 to 40 minutes including preparation, baking, and cooling. It makes up to 8 servings.

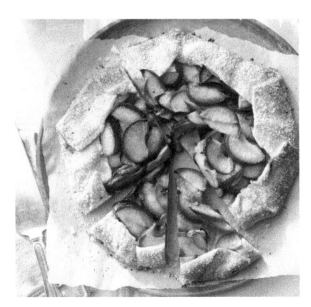

- Large egg (1) only egg white

- Pie crust (refrigerated)

- Fresh plums (sliced); 3 and a half cups

- Coarse sugar (1 teaspoon and 3 tablespoons)

- Cornstarch; 1 tablespoon

- Crystallized ginger (chopped); 2 teaspoons

- Water; 1 tablespoon

Preheat the oven to 400°. Unroll crust on a work surface. Then roll it in a 12-inches circle. Transfer to a baking sheet covered with parchment.

Toss the plums in a wide bowl with 3 spoonsful of cornstarch and sugar. Arrange crust plums up to about 2 in. Of the edges; sprinkle the ginger over. Fold the edge of the crust over the prunes and pleat as you go.

Whisk egg white and water in a small bowl; sprinkle over folded crust. Sprinkle of extra sugar.

Bake for 20 to 25 minutes, until crust is golden brown. Cool on a wire rack, on a tray. Serve warm, or at ambient temperature.

4. Cake - Pear Bundt

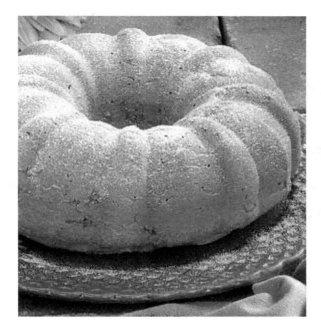

The cake gives you around 15 to 16 servings using the following ingredients. Moreover, it takes about one hour including preparation, baking, and cooling.

- Sliced pears (sugar reduced) 1 can

- White cake mix; 1 Packet

- Large eggs (2) egg whites only

- Large egg; 1, whole

- Confectioner sugar; 2 teaspoons

Drain pears and set aside the syrup; chop pears. In a big cup, put the pears and syrup; add the cake mixture, the egg whites, and the butter. Beat 30 seconds on low speed. Beat 4 minutes on high.

Coat them in a 10-inches tube pan with cooking spray and flour residue. Add the ingredients.

Bake at 350 ° until 50 to 55 minutes comes out clean with a toothpick inserted in the middle. Give it 10 minutes to cool completely before transferring from pan to wire rack. Dust it using the confectioner sugar.

However, you can use other fruits as well as frozen strawberries with a white cake mix to work well!

5. Banana Raspberry Soft Serve (ice cream)

The total time this soft serve takes is around 10 to 15 minutes plus cooling. The following ingredients can make 2 cups easily.

- Ripe bananas; 4 medium-sized
- Fat-free yogurt; Half cup
- Maple syrup; 1 to 2 tablespoons
- Unsweetened Raspberries (frozen); Half cup
- Raspberries/blueberries (fresh); optional

Thinly slice the bananas; transfer to something like a large plastic resealable freezer bag. Set slices together in a layer and then freeze them overnight.

Pulse the bananas until finely diced in a food processor. Add milk, raspberries and maple syrup. Then process until smooth, scrubbing sides as necessary. Serve straight away, add fresh berries if you wish.

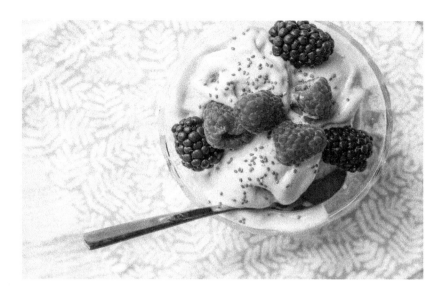

Chocolate-Peanut Butter: Substitute for the raspberries; 2 tablespoons of each peanut butter or baking cocoa; continue as instructed.

6. Butterscotch Pumpkin Gingerbread Trifle

It requires 40 minutes for preparation and baking requires around 35 to 40 minutes. Cooling takes extra time. It makes up to 16 servings.

- Gingerbread cookie or cake mix (1 packet)

- Fat-free or low-fat milk; 4 cups

- Ground cinnamon (1 teaspoon)

- Butterscotch pudding (sugar-free) mix; 4 packets 1 oz. each

- Ground ginger; ¼ teaspoon

- Ground allspice; ¼ teaspoon

- Ground nutmeg; ¼ teaspoon

- Pumpkin; 1 can, 15 oz.

- Whipped topping (low-fat, frozen) 12 oz.

Prepare and bake the gingerbread mix according to cake packaging directions. Then, cool it.

Break the cake into crumbles; save the crumbs for 1/4 cup. Whisk the butter, pudding mixtures, and spices in a wide bowl until the mixture thickens, around 2 minutes. Stir in the pumpkin.

In a qt of 3–1/2. trifle or glass cup, 1/4 layer of cake crumbs, 1/2 pumpkin mixture, 1/4 of the cake crumbs, and 1/2 whipped topping; repeat the layering. Top with crumbs that are reserved. Chill once done.

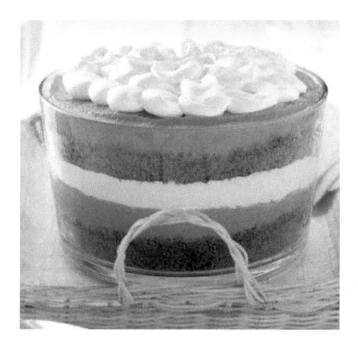

7. Raspberry Chocolate Cheesecake

This cheesecake takes around 25 to 30 minutes for preparation then it takes some time to cool off. You can prepare 12 servings using the following ingredients.

- Melted butter; 2 tablespoons

- Crumbs of Graham Crackers; ¾ cup

- Gelatin (unflavored); 1 envelope

- Coldwater; 1 cup

- Half cup sugar

- Baking cocoa; ¼ cup

- Semisweet chocolate (chopped); 4 oz.

- Cream cheese (fat-free or low-fat); 4 packets 8 oz. each

- Vanilla extract; 2 teaspoons

- Fresh raspberries; 2 cups

- Sugar substitute; 1 cup sugar

Combine cracker crumbs and butter; push to a grated 9 inches pan. Bake for 8-10 minutes at 375 °, or until light brown. Cool it off.

Sprinkle the gelatin over cold water in a medium saucepan for filling; let stand for 1 minute. Heat over low heat, stirring until the gelatin dissolves completely. Stir in the semi-sweet candy, once cooled.

Beat the cream cheese, sugar replacement, and butter in a large bowl until they are smooth. Gradually substitute the blend of sugar and cocoa. Fill them in coffee. Pour over the crust; cool for 2-3 hours or until solid.

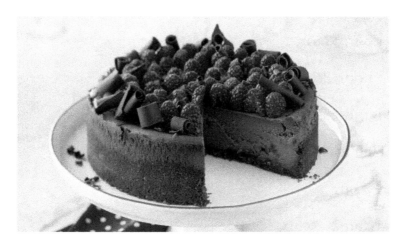

Set raspberries on a cheesecake. Loosen the cake from the pan using a knife carefully.

8. Chocolate chip cookies – Browned Butter

Butter shifts from nutty and sweet to salty and easily charred, but make careful to remove the pan from the fire until it becomes amber-colored. Make sure the cookie sheet is absolutely clean before beginning the next batch to prevent cookies from spreading.

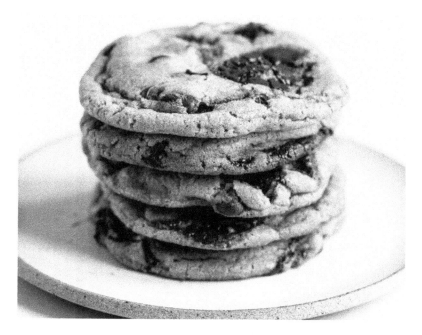

- Unsalted Butter; 6 tablespoons

- Canola oil; 2 tablespoons

- All-purpose flour; 5.6 oz.

- Whole-wheat flour; 3.3 oz.

- Baking powder; 1 teaspoon

- Kosher salt; Half teaspoon

- Brown sugar; ¾ cup

- Granulated sugar; 2/3 cup

- Vanilla extract; Half teaspoon

- Large eggs (2), slightly beaten

- Chocolate chips (semisweet); Half cup

- Hershey's Chocolate chips (dark); 1/3 cup

Preheat the oven to 375°.

Heat the butter over medium heat in a small saucepan; cook for 5 minutes or until brown. Take off heat; add oil. Put aside to freshen up.

Weigh or gently spoon flours into dry cups of measurement; level with a knife. Stir with a fork, mix flours, baking powder, and salt. Put the butter and sugar mixture in a bowl; beat at medium speed with a mixer until mixed. Add eggs and vanilla; beat till it's blended. Add flour mixture, beat at low velocity until just mixed. Add chocolate chips.

Pour 2 inches on baking trays lined with a waxed paper by even spoonful. Bake for 12 minutes or when cookie bottoms only start to get brown. Then cool them a bit.

9. Chocolate Coconut Cupcakes

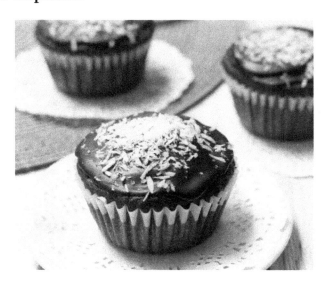

These cupcakes require 20 minutes for preparation, 30 minutes for baking, and then some time to cool off. You can make around a dozen cupcakes.

- Egg whites (large eggs); 6

- All-purpose flour; 2/3 cup

- Baking cocoa; ¼ cup

- Baking powder; Half teaspoon

- Sugar; 1 to 1 1/3 cup

- Almond extract; 1 teaspoon

- Cream of tartar; 1 teaspoon

- Salt; ¼ teaspoon

- Shredded Coconut (sweetened); 1 cup

- Confectioner Sugar

Preheat your oven to 350°.

Put the egg whites in a bowl. Line 18 cups of cupcake muffin liners. Mix the flour, baking powder, cocoa, and 1 cup of sugar.

Add almond extract, tartar cream, and salt to egg whites; beat at medium velocity until soft peaks develop. Gradually add the remaining sugar, 1 teaspoon at a time, and beat before the sugar is dissolved. Continue to beat until stiff glittering peaks emerge. Gradually add in flour mixture, one and a half cup at a time. Fold softly in a cocoon.

Fill two-thirds of prepared cups completely. Bake for 30 to 35 minutes, until the top is crisp.

Wait in pans for 10 minutes before transferring to wire racks; cool the cupcakes completely. Dust it off using confectioner sugar if needed.

10. Apple Pie (No Bake)

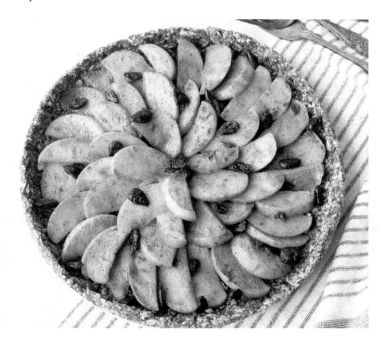

Apples are distributed often during the year and that is something you should take advantage of. This pie takes about 20-25 minutes for preparation. Then, it takes time to cool off. The following ingredients can prepare up to 8 servings.

- Tart apples; medium-sized; 5; sliced and peeled

- Lemon gelatin (sugar-free); 1 packet

- Ground cinnamon; Half teaspoon

- Ground nutmeg; ¼ teaspoon

- Water (divided); 1 and ¾ cups

- Sugar-free Vanilla Pudding mix

- Chopped Nuts; Half cup

- Crust made using Graham Crackers; 1 piece

- Whipped topping

Mix the gelatin, nutmeg, cinnamon, and water in a large saucepan. Stir in apples; put to a simmer. Reduce heat; boil, cover, for around 5 minutes, until apples are tender.

Mix pudding mixture and remaining water in a bowl; stir in apple mixture. Cook for about 1 minute, stirring occasionally until thickened. Take off heat; stir in the nuts. Remove it from the pan.

Refrigerate the pie two hours before eating. Serve with whipped topping if desired.

11. Frozen Yogurt and Berry Popsicle Swirls

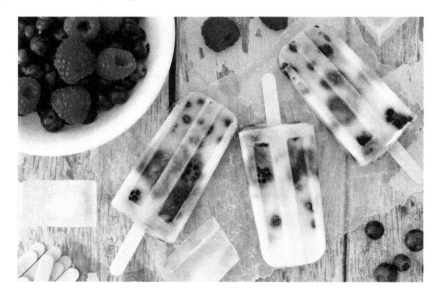

Preparation for these swirls requires 15 to 20 minutes. It is a good and healthy way to ease your ice cream or sugar cravings. After preparation, it takes time to freeze. You can make 10 popsicles with the following ingredients.

- Fresh berries; 1 cup

- Fat-free Greek Yogurt; 2 ¾ cups

- Paper or Plastic cups; 10

- Water; ¼ cup

- Sugar; 2 tablespoons

- Pop sticks (wooden); 10

Every cup is filled with around 1/4 cup yogurt. In a food processor, put the berries, water, and sugar; pulse until the berries are finely chopped. spoon berry mixture into each cup. Stir softly and play with a pop button.

Foil the cups from the top; drop through foil the pop sticks. Freeze them until they are solid.

For Frozen Yogurt Clementine Swirls: Replace 1 cup of clementine seeded segments and 1/4 cup of orange juice for sugar, berries, and water; follow the instructions.

12. Root Beer Pie

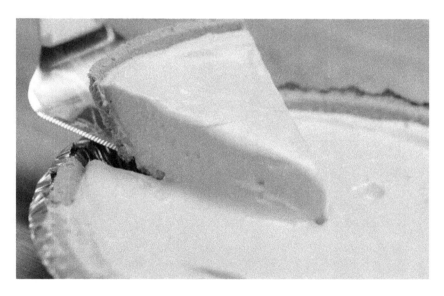

For its preparation, you will need 15 to 20 minutes. You need the following ingredients for this pie.

- Crust; Graham Cracker

- Vanilla Pudding Mix; 1 packet

- Whipped topping (low-fat); frozen

- Diet root beer; ¾ cup

- Fat-free or low-fat milk; Half cup

- Cherries (optional)

Set aside and cool for garnish the whipped coating. Whisk the root beer, sugar, and pudding mixture in a wide bowl for 2 minutes. Fold the leftover whipped topping in two. Apply on the crust of graham cracker.

Place over tar left whipped coating. Freeze at least eight hours, or overnight.

Garnish the reserved whipped topping over each serving; if desired, top with a cherry maraschino.

13. Jelly and Peanut Butter Sandwich Cookies

Peanut butter cookies form the ideal basis for spreading a coating of delicious strawberry. Serve some delicious cookies as an afternoon snack or a surprise warm lunchbox.

- Soft margarine; ¼ cup

- Peanut butter (creamy); no sugar; ¼ cup

- Sweetener (calorie-free); Half cup

- Sugar; ¼ cup

- Egg whites (2); Large eggs

- Vanilla Extract; 1 teaspoon

- All-purpose Flour; 1 ¾ cup

- Baking soda; 1 teaspoon

- Salt, 1/8 teaspoon

- Cooking spray

- Strawberry spread (low-sugar); ¾ cup

Preheat the oven to 350°.

Beat peanut butter and butter until creamy, with a mixer at medium speed. Gradually add sugar and sweetener, and beat well. Then add the vanilla and the egg whites. In a bowl, combine the flour, salt, and soda, and stir well. Gradually add the flour to the creamed mixture and beat well.

Dough form into 40 balls, 1-inch each. Put the balls with a distance of 2 inches between them on cooking spray-coated baking sheets. Use a glass or anything flat to flatten the cookies into 2-inch circles. Bake for 8 to 9 minutes at 350 °, or until lightly browned. Cool on pans; cut, and let cool down on wire racks.

Spread strawberry on each of the 20 cookies at the bottom; top with remaining cookies.

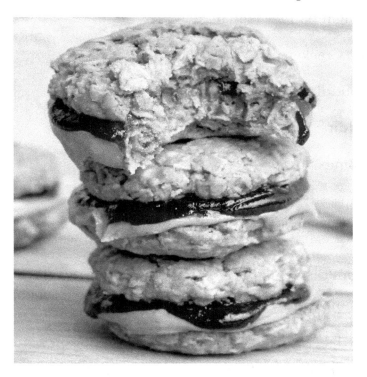

14. Pudding Pie

For someone with diabetes, this pie is surely what you need to quench your sugar cravings. It takes 20 minutes for preparation. You can make 8 servings using the following ingredients.

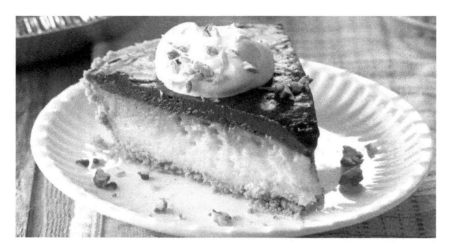

- Fat-free milk; 4 cups

- Vanilla pudding mix; 1 oz. (sugar-free)

- Crust; Graham Cracker

- Butterscotch pudding mix; 1 oz. (sugar-free)

- Chocolate pudding mix; 1 oz. (sugar-free)

- Whipped topping

- Chopped pecans

Whisk the milk and the vanilla pudding mixture for 2 minutes. Spread over crust.

Whisk butterscotch pudding mixture and milk in another bowl for 2 minutes. Carefully spoon over the top of the coffee, thinly distributed.

Whisk the remaining 1-1/3 cups of milk and chocolate pudding mixture into a separate bowl for 2 minutes. Spread carefully over top. Refrigerate at least 30 minutes when you are done. Serve with whipped toppings and pecans if needed.

15. Chocolate Cupcakes

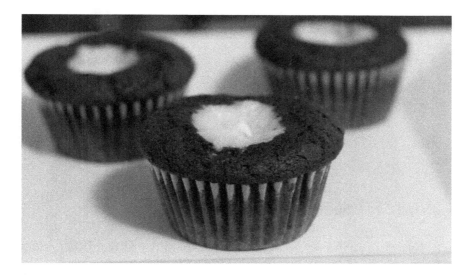

Inside these chocolate cupcakes is a secret, delicious filling of coconut and ricotta cheese. These cupcakes require 20 minutes for preparation and around 30 minutes for baking. Then, it takes time to cool off. You can make a dozen cupcakes with the following ingredients.

- Egg whites; 2 large eggs

- Large egg (1)

- Applesauce (unsweetened); 1/3 cup

- Vanilla extract; 1 teaspoon

- All-purpose flour; 1 to 1 ¼ cups

- Sugar; 1 cup

- Baking cocoa; 1/3 cup

- Baking soda; ½ teaspoon

- Buttermilk; ¾ cup

To prepare the filling for the cupcakes, you need:

- Ricotta cheese (low-fat); 1 cup

- Sugar; ¼ cup

- Egg white; 1 large egg

- Shredded coconut (sweetened); 1/3 cup

- Almond or coconut extract; Half teaspoon

- Confectioner Sugar

Preheat your oven to 350°. Coat 18 muffin cups with cooking oil.

Beat 4 ingredients first, until well combined. Whisk together flour, cocoa, sugar, and baking soda in another bowl; slowly beat alternately with buttermilk into an egg mixture.

Beat the ricotta cheese, sugar, and white egg until combined for filling. Stir in coconut.

Fill the muffin cups using batter but use only half. Fill your filling into the middle of each cupcake by the tablespoonfuls; cover with remaining batter.

Bake for 28 to 33 minutes and wait for the toothpick inserted in the cupcake to come out neat. Transfer after 10 minutes on wire racks before removing from the pans. Dust it using confectioners' sugar.

15. Wheat and Seed Bread

This bread is expensive to make than normal loaves of bread, so for a couple of days, I recommend you slice and freeze any that you won't use. Despite the high fat and protein content, it is full. I don't need insulin for that sandwich, but it's not the same for everybody. For anything that includes a touch of carbohydrate, I require insulin so I realized that the protein and fat in the ingredients would help offset the carbohydrates in

the ingredients, but I was also happily shocked that I didn't need insulin at all. No sugar, no hypo- threat. This bread is good not only for people with diabetes but for everyone.

- Almond flour; 80 grams

- Coconut flour; 30 grams

- Psyllium Husk; 20 grams

- Melted Butter; 30 grams

- Buttermilk; 1 cup

- Mixed seeds

- Baking powder; ¼ teaspoon

- Bread soda; Half teaspoon

- Flaxseed; 50 grams

- Wheat Bran; 30 grams

Preheat your oven to 180°C. Line a one-pound loaf tin with baking parchment paper or you can also use a liner if you want.

Sieve into a cup the coconut and almond or ground almond, bread soda, and baking powder.

Add the rest of the dry ingredients, also the seeds.

Combine the buttermilk, eggs and melted butter in a bowl, then mix.

Build a well with the dry ingredients in the middle. Add the liquid and stir to mix both the dry ingredients and the liquid in a circular motion. Don't over-mix them. A loose batter is what you need as your mixture.

Put your mixture into a lined loaf pan. Place first 15 minutes in the preheated oven, then lower it to 150 ° C. Bake for another 25 minutes or until the bread is baked. You will see the bread rising from the edges of the pan. The time taken to cook depends on your oven.

Allow the bread to cool on a rack. The bread can be kept for 3 to 4 days in the freezer, although the day it is cooked it needs to be frozen if you decide to preserve it longer.

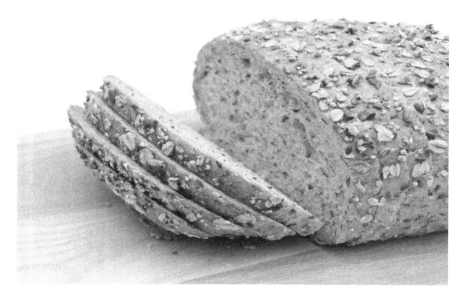

16. Coffee Cupcakes

Such chocolatey cupcakes are kept on the lighter side using low-fat whipped icing to dust them. You should substitute the prune puree with unsweetened applesauce if you want.

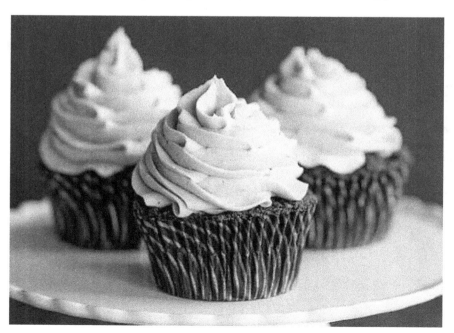

It takes about 15 minutes for preparation. For baking, the cupcakes need 20 minutes. Then, cooling requires extra time!

- Eggs (2)

- All-purpose flour; 2 cups

- Baking cocoa; Half cup

- Baking soda; 1 teaspoon

- Salt; Half teaspoon

- Hot water; Half cup

- Coffee Granules (instant); ¼ cup

- Baby food; Half cup

- Canola oil; ¼ cup

- Vanilla extract; 2 teaspoons

- Whipped topping (low-fat)

- Baking cocoa (additional)

Combine the cocoa, flour, baking soda, sugar, and salt in a bowl. Dissolve the coffee in hot water. Whisk the whites, baby meal, butter, espresso, and coffee mixture in a big pot. Gradually mix in dry ingredients until moist.

Fill up two-thirds muffin cups. Bake for 18 to 20 minutes at 350 °, or until a toothpick comes out clean. Wait for about 10 minutes and then you can remove the cupcakes from pans to wire racks.

Shortly before eating, brush with chocolate and fill cupcakes with whipped icing. Store the leftovers in a refrigerator.

17. Chocolate Banana Cake

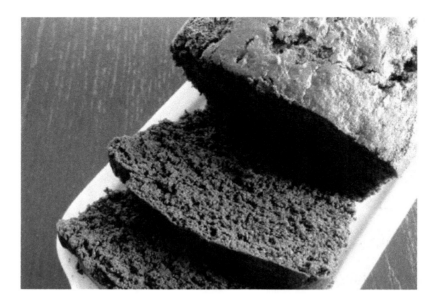

This chocolate light-as-air cake has a yummy banana flavor. It's delicious as it is, so you can dress it up with nuts or soft frostings as well. The cake requires 15 minutes for the preparation. It takes 25 minutes for baking and then it cools down. This cake has about 12 servings.

- Soft butter; 1/3 cup

- Sugar substitute; ¾ cup

- Brown sugar; 1/3 cup

- Vanilla extract; 2 teaspoons

- Large eggs (2)

- Water; Half cup

- All-purpose flour; 1 1/3 cup

- Milk powder (zero fat); Half cup

- Baking cocoa; 3 tablespoons

- Baking powder; 1 teaspoon

- Baking soda; Half teaspoon

- Salt; Half teaspoon

- Ripe bananas; mashed; 1 cup

- Confectioner sugar

Preheat the oven to 375°. Coat a 9 inches square pan using cooking spray.

Mix butter, a substitute for sugar, and brown sugar until light and fluffy. Then add the coffee and whites, beat well as you add each ingredient, one at a time. Stir the water in. Whisk together flour, cocoa, milk powder, baking soda, baking powder, and salt. Keep it mixing until you get a creamy texture. Stir in the bananas.

Switch to the prepared pan. Then bake for 23- to minutes before a toothpick inserted in the middle comes out clean and the cake starts to fall from the sides of the oven. Cool down on a wire rack. Dust it with confectioners' sugar.

18. Sour Cream Cake

This is a lighter cake recipe with the traditional one's flavor. Reduced-fat sour cream, without too many calories, contains moisture and flavor.

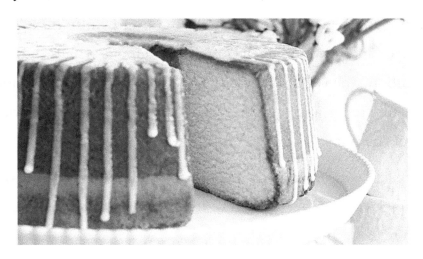

- Large eggs (3)

- Cooking spray

- Breadcrumbs; 3 tablespoons

- Cake flour; 4 cups

- Salt; ¼ teaspoon

- Sour cream (light); 1 and a half cup

- Baking soda; 1 teaspoon

- Butter; ¾ cup

- Sugar; 2 ¾ cups

- Vanilla extract; 2 teaspoons

- Lemon juice (fresh); 2 tablespoons

Preheat the oven to 350°.

Coat a 10 inches pan using cooking spray and dust it with breadcrumbs.

Lightly add flour in dry cups and level them using a knife. Combine flour and salt; mix with a whisk. Bring sour cream and baking soda together; stir well. Layer butter in a wide bowl; beat medium-speed using a mixer until light and fluffy. Gradually incorporate cinnamon and sugar, and beat until well combined. Remove whites, 1 at a time, then beat well with any addition. Then add some juice; beat for 30 seconds. Now, add flour mixture to sugar mixture, mixing at a low level, starting and finishing with flour mixture, and with the mixture of sour cream.

Spoon batter in ready pan. Bake for 1 hour and 10 minutes at 350 °, or until a center inserted wooden pick comes out clean. Cool for 10 minutes and then remove it from the pan. Fully cool on rack wire.

19. Crackle Cookies

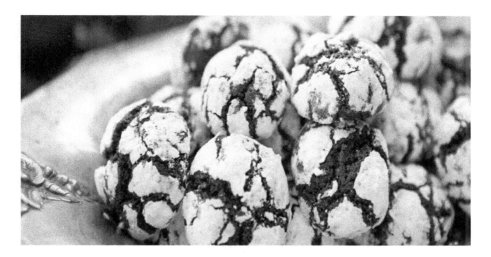

Without any guilt, you should treat yourself to one or two of those crackle cookies. It takes 20 minutes for preparation. And you can easily make 2 dozen cookies using the following ingredients.

- Sugar; 2/3 cup

- Large egg (1)

- Canola oil; ¼ cup

- Molasses; 1/3 cup

- Whole-wheat flour; 2 cups

- Baking soda; 1 teaspoon

- Ground cinnamon; 1 teaspoon

- Ground ginger; ¼ teaspoon

- Ground cloves; ¼ teaspoon

- Salt; Half teaspoon

- Confectioner Sugar; 1 tablespoon

Beat oil and sugar in a bowl, until mixed. Place in molasses and eggs. Combine the starch, baking soda, salt, cinnamon, cloves, and ginger; introduce the sugar mixture slowly, and blend properly. Refrigerate and cover for at least 2 hours.

Preheat the oven to 350°. Dough to 1-inch balls; roll the balls in confectioner sugar. Place the balls with 2 inches distance between them on a spray-coated baking sheet; partially flatten. Bake for seven to nine minutes or until completed. To cool off, place it on wire racks.

A single cookie contains approx. 77 calories.

20. Pudding Cookie Sandwiches

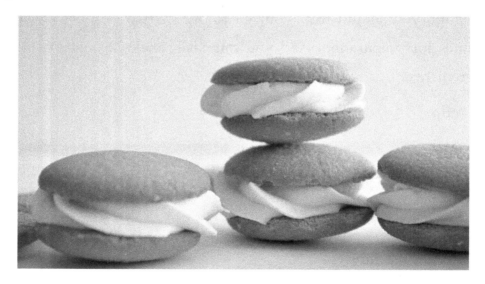

Preparation for these cookies requires 20 minutes. You can make more than 2 dozen cookies with the following ingredients.

- Fat-free or low-fat milk; 1 to 2 cups

- Chocolate pudding mix; sugar-free; 1.4 oz.

- Whipped topping; low-fat; frozen; 8 oz.

- Marshmallows; 1 cup

- Chocolate wafers; 9 oz.

Whisk the milk and pudding mix for 2 minutes to fill; allow it to stand for 2 minutes. Fold in topping and then marshmallows.

Place around 2 tablespoons onto the bottom of a wafer for each sandwich; cover with another wafer. Place the sandwiches in sealed pots.

Freeze up for around 3 hours. Remove from the freezer before 5 minutes to serve.

21. Chocolate Hazelnut Popsicles

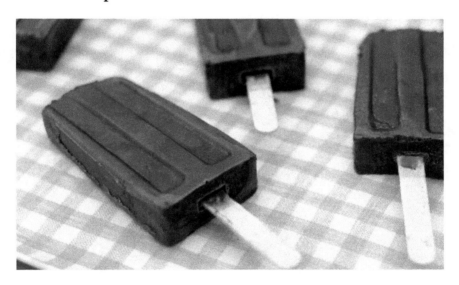

If you love Nutella as I do, this is the thing for you. You need 10 minutes for the preparation of these popsicles. And you can make 8 of these using the following ingredients.

- Nutella; 1/3 cup

- Popsicle molds or paper/plastic cups; 8

- Soy milk (vanilla); 1 cup

- Fat-free milk; Half cup

- Greek yogurt (vanilla) fat-free; ¾ cup

- Pop sticks (wooden)

Place Nutella, yogurt, and milk in a blender; cover it and blend it until smooth. Pour into paper cups or popsicle molds. Cover the molds with holders. If you are using cups, cover with foil and then insert sticks through the foil. Freeze until solid.

One popsicle contains approx. 94 to 95 calories.

22. Chocolate Cheesecake

This cheesecake appears indulgent, it is a lightened-up variety so you should feel confident about feeding your mates. It takes 30 minutes for preparation and 40 minutes for baking. The cooling time in between is extra. You can get 12 servings per cake.

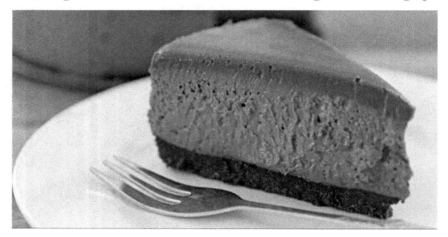

- Cottage Cheese; 2%; 2 cups

- Chocolate wafers (crushed); 1 cup

- Low-fat cream cheese; 1 packet; 8 oz.

- Sugar; Half cup

- Dash salt

- Vanilla extract; 1 tablespoon

- Large eggs (2); slightly beaten

- Egg white (1); a large egg

- Melted then cooled bittersweet chocolate; 2 oz.

- Raspberries are optional

Fill a strainer with cheesecloth having four layers or a coffee filter; position it over a pot. Put the cottage cheese in a strainer; refrigerate for 1 hour. Bring in a 9 inches pan at a double thickness of foil, tightly seal foil around the pan. Coat with a cooking spray inside of the pan. Push down broken wafers, then 1-inch to the upper side.

Preheat the oven to 350°. Process drained cheese in a food processor until it is smooth. Attach cinnamon, sugar, and cream cheese; heat until combined. Shift to a bowl and then add the egg white, eggs, and coffee. In a bowl, remove 1 cup batter; mix in molten chocolate.

Drop the batter on your crust. Place chocolate cake over simple batter. Cut with a knife to run into water. Transfer to a bigger pan. Then add hot water to a pan.

Bake until the center is set and top appears. Bake it for around 40 minutes. Switch off oven; partially open the screen. Give your cheesecake 30 minutes to cool down.

Remove the water pan and then remove foil. Loosen cheesecake sides with a knife; cool down for approx. 30 minutes on a wire rack. Refrigerate overnight and keep it covered.

You can top it with raspberries or anything you want!

23. Fruit Pizza

There is nothing better than a dessert that you can eat without any guilt, particularly when it is surmounted with delicious, colorful fruit. It requires 25 minutes for preparation and extra time for cooling. Then, you need 10 minutes for baking and more extra time for cooling.

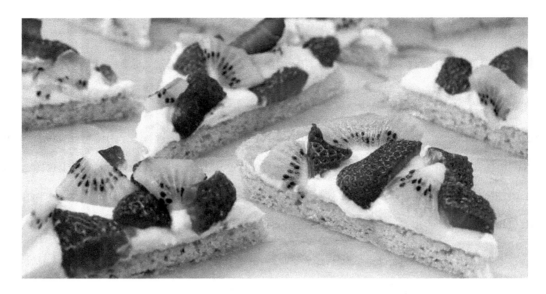

- All-purpose flour; 1 cup

- Butter; Half cup

- Confectioner sugar; ¼ cup

To prepare the glaze for your fruit pizza, you need the following ingredients.

- Cornstarch; 5 teaspoons

- Pineapple juice (unsweetened); 1 ¼ cups

- Lemon juice; 1 teaspoon

For the preparation of your fruit pizza topping, you require the following ingredients.

- Cream cheese (fat-free or low-fat); 8 oz.

- Sugar; 1/3 cup

- Vanilla extract; 1 teaspoon

- Fresh strawberries; 2 cups

- Fresh blueberries; 1 cup

- Oranges; 1 can

You can add more fruit if you like!

Preheat the oven to 350°. In a bowl, mix confectioners' sugar and flour; add butter until you get a crumbly texture. Press it in an ungreased pizza pan (12 inches). Bake until it gets light brown, for about 10 to 12 minutes. Cool it completely.

In a saucepan, mix glaze ingredients and keep mixing until it gets smooth. Then bring the mixture to a boil. Cook it until thick for approx. 2 minutes. Cool it.

Take a bowl, beat sugar, vanilla, and cream cheese until smooth. Now, spread it over the crust. You can top it with berries or mandarin oranges. And drizzle it with glaze. Keep it refrigerated until its cold and firm.

24. Chocolate Chip and Banana Cookies

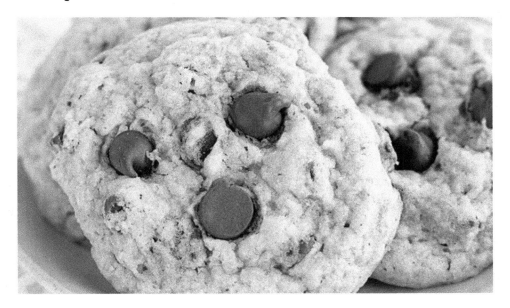

Such fluffy cookies with banana have a cakelike feel and plenty of taste that everybody seems to enjoy. You need 20 minutes for the preparation and then, baking requires 15 to 20 minutes. You can make more than 2 dozen cookies with the following ingredients.

- All-purpose flour; 1 ¼ cup

- Softened butter; 1/3 cup

- Large egg (1)

- Ripe banana (mashed); Half cup

- Vanilla extract; Half teaspoon

- Baking powder; 1 teaspoon

- Salt; ¼ teaspoon

- Baking soda; 1/8 teaspoon

- Chocolate chips (semisweet); 1 cup

In a bowl, mix butter and sugar until it gets fluffy. Beat in the egg, banana, and vanilla. Mix the flour with baking powder, salt, and baking soda; slowly add to the creamed mixture and mix it well. Then, stir in chocolate chips.

Drop the batter by tablespoonfuls with a distance of approx. 2 inches in between them on the baking sheets that you sprayed with cooking spray. Now, bake them at 350°; 13 to 16 minutes or wait until they are light brown. Cool them down on wire racks.

Tips:

Stir 1/2 cup of diced toasted walnuts or pecans into the batter for additional flavor. Toast almonds, bake for 5 to 10 minutes in a pan at 350 ° in an oven, or roast over low heat in a skillet until well browned.

Use ripe ones to produce the maximum taste when baking with bananas. Layer bananas

and an egg, mango, tomato or peach in a brown paper bag and leave it on your counter if you can spare a day or two. It will collect the fruit's ethylene gas, and speed the maturing cycle. To ripen bananas much quicker, place them on a baking sheet in their peels, and steam them up for 15 to 20 minutes in a 250° oven.

25. Strawberry Cheesecake – Choco-topped

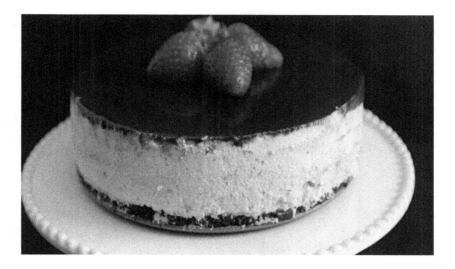

Creamy and soft, this beautiful dessert is something perfect for a summer party. It takes 35 minutes for preparation and then extra time for cooling. Another 10 minutes for baking and extra time for cooling it again. You can get 12 servings per cake.

- Crumbs – Graham Crackers; 1 ¼ cups

- Melted butter; ¼ cup

- Unflavored Gelatin; 2 envelopes

- Coldwater; Half cup

- Frozen Strawberries (unsweetened); 16 oz.

- Cream cheese (fat-free); 8 oz. 2 packets

- Cottage cheese (fat-free); 1 cup

- Sugar substitute; ¾ cup

- Whipped topping (low-fat); 8 oz.

- Topping (ice cream) chocolate; Half cup

- Fresh strawberries; 1 cup

Preheat the oven to 350°.

Mix the butter and crumbs; press downwards and 1-inch upwards in a 9 inches pan sprayed with cooking mist. Place on a sheet to bake. Bake for about 10 minutes, until set. Cool down on a wire rack.

Sprinkle gelatin in cold water in a small saucepan and then allow it to stand for 1 minute. Heat over low pressure, stir until the gelatin is dissolved completely; remove from fire.

Where appropriate, hull strawberries in a food processor. Empty it in a bowl. Then in a food processor, add cream cheese, cottage cheese, and substitute sugar, process it until it gets creamy and smooth. Gradually add gelatin mixture while it is being processed. Pureed strawberries are added; blend it well. Pass to a bowl; fold overtopping in 2 cups. Spread it on the crust. Cover, refrigerate for 2 to 3 hours.

Loosen the sides of the cheesecake using a knife and then remove the rim. You can use chocolate topping when serving or strawberries or whipped topping.

26. Cloud Bread

Try the Cloud Bread the next time you're having a pizza or some other meal containing slices of bread. Cloud Bread is a fully gluten-free option to low-carb, low-calorie, and low-fat food. It's a healthy choice and tastes good! You can also make pizza on a cloud bread!

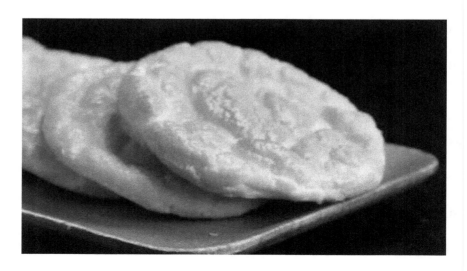

- Eggs (3)

- Softened cream cheese; 3 tablespoons

- Sugar; 1 teaspoon

- Cream of tartar; ¼ teaspoon

Preheat the oven to 300 degrees F. Then, coat 2 baking sheets using cooking spray.

In a bowl, mix cream cheese, sugar and egg yolks until smooth.

In another bowl, combine egg whites with tartar cream; beat with a high-speed electric mixer until fluffy and steep peaks shape. Gently fold the egg yolk mixture into a blend of egg white until well-integrated. Spoon mixture on baking sheets into 10 rounds.

Bake it for 25 to 30 minutes approx., or until it is golden brown. Let it cool for 5 minutes and then transfer it to a wire rack allowing it to cool completely.

Tips:

How to Store Cloud Bread: An airtight container is the best option if you want to store this bread.

How to Freeze Cloud Bread: Freeze after allowing it to cool. Remember that after being frozen the bread takes on a lighter texture.

What to Eat with Cloud Bread: This bread is a replacement for your regular bread. You can either eat it just like that or you can eat it with any spread. You can also make a sandwich using this bread. You can also make a pizza with this bread.

27. Peanut Butter Balls – No-Bake

Such peanut butter oatmeal balls are great for road trips and do not stick to your hands. They make a good snack! It takes only 10 minutes to prepare!

- Peanut Butter (chunky); 1/3 cup

- Honey; ¼ cup

- Vanilla extract; Half teaspoon

- Milk powder; 1/3 cup (fat-free)

- Oats (quick-cooking); 1/3 cup

- Crumbs; Graham Crackers; 2 tablespoons

Mix the honey and vanilla with peanut butter in a bowl. Stir in the oats, graham cracker crumbs, and the milk powder. Shape the mixture into small 1-inch balls. Now, cover and refrigerate before serving.

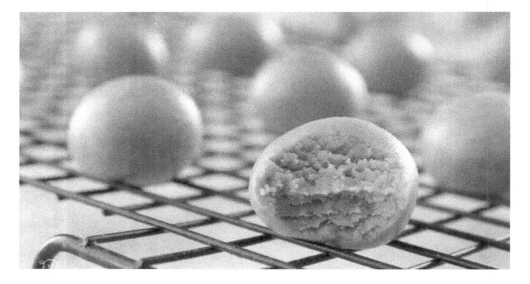

28. Orange Food Cake

Thanks to a touch of orange flavor swirled through every slice, a simple angel food cake is a heavenly indulgence. The preparation for this cake requires about 25 minutes and 30 minutes for baking. You can get 16 servings per cake.

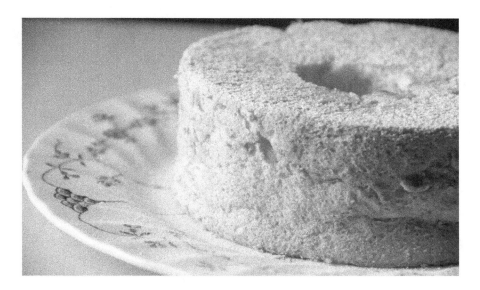

- Egg whites; 12 eggs

- All-purpose flour; 1 cup

- Sugar; 1 ¾ cup

- Cream of tartar; 1 ½ teaspoon

- Salt; Half teaspoon

- Almond extract; 1 teaspoon

- Vanilla extract; 1 teaspoon

- Orange zest (grated); 1 teaspoon

- Orange extract; 1 teaspoon

- Food color (red); 6 drops

- Food color (yellow); 6 drops

Put egg whites in a bowl; allow it to stand at room temperature for about 30 minutes. Mix flour and sugar together twice and then set it aside.

To egg whites, add salt, cream of tartar, and vanilla and almond extracts; beat at medium speed until soft peaks develop. Then, add remaining sugar, around 2 teaspoons at a time, beating fast to create sharp, shiny peaks and dissolve sugar. Then, add in flour mixture, one and a half cup at a time.

Gently pour half of the batter into a 10 inches ungreased pan. Stir in the orange extract, orange zest, and the food color if necessary, to the remaining batter. Spoon orange batter gently over white batter. Cut with a knife into all sides to shake the orange and draw out the air pockets.

Bake at 375° for about 30 to 35 minutes on the oven's lowest rack. Bake it until it is light brown and its top appears to be dry. Then invert pan quickly and cool it for almost one hour.

Remove the cake using a knife to loosen the sides and put it on a serving plate!

29. Meringue Cookies – Vanilla

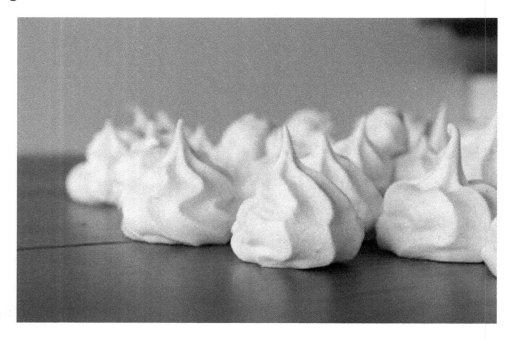

This cookie is sweet, airy and the ultimate fat-free dessert to help fight a desire for sweets. Ingredient preparation requires 20 minutes, and baking and standing require 40 minutes.

You can make approx. 5 dozen cookies with these ingredients.

- Egg whites (large); 3 eggs

- Vanilla extract; 1 ½ teaspoon

- Cream of tartar; ¼ teaspoon

- Sugar; 2/3 cup

- Dash salt

Pour egg whites in a bowl and allow them to stand for 30 minutes at room temperature. Preheat the oven to 250°. Then, add cream of tartar, salt, and vanilla to the egg whites and beat the mixture until it gives a foam-like texture. Then, slowly add sugar and keep beating it high after each tablespoon is added until all the sugar dissolves. Keep beating it until it takes the form for approx. 7 minutes.

Cut a small hole in a pastry bag tip then insert a # 32-star tip. Fill the piping bag with your meringue mixture. Make cookie shapes using the tip on your piping bag, keep them small in size and at a distance from each other on the paper-lined baking sheets.

Bake for 40 to 45 minutes. Turn the oven off; keep the meringues in the oven for 1 hour and keep the oven door close. Clear from the oven; refrigerate fully on baking sheets. Cut the meringues from paper; place them at room temperature in an airtight container.

Tips:

- Room-temperature and old eggs make better meringues.

- On a dry day, it is better to make these cookies because on rainy or humid days they absorb moisture easily and become sticky.

30. Applesauce Brownies

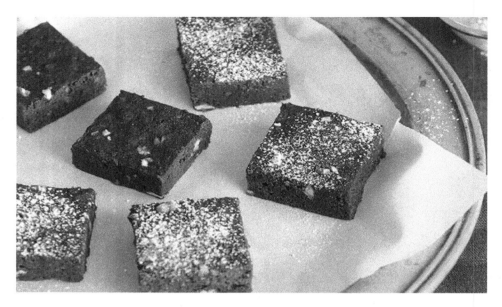

These brownies are easy to make and they taste good too. The preparation time for these brownie ingredients is 15 minutes approximately. Baking requires around 25 minutes along with cooling the brownies.

- Softened Butter; ¼ cup

- Sugar; ¾ cup

- Large egg

- All-purpose flour; 1 cup

- Baking cocoa; 1 tablespoon

- Baking soda; Half teaspoon

- Ground cinnamon; Half teaspoon

- Applesauce; 1 cup

For the topping, you need:

- Chocolate chips; Half cup

- Pecans or walnuts (chopped); Half cup

- Sugar; 1 tablespoon

Mix sugar and butter in a bowl. Beat an egg in. Then, mix the flour with cocoa, cinnamon, and baking soda. Then slowly add it to the creamy mixture and mix it well. Add in applesauce. Drop into an 8 inches baking pan (square) sprayed with cooking spray.

Combine the topping ingredients and sprinkle it over batter. Bake your brownies at 350° for about 25 minutes or keep check until the toothpick in the center comes out neat. Let it cool and then cut it in squares!

31. Oatmeal Cookies

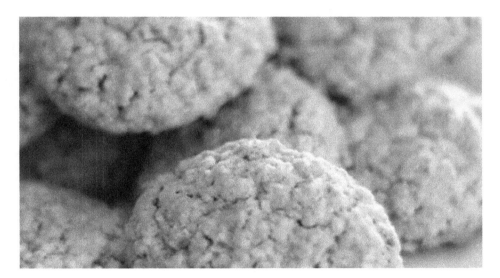

You need 35 to 40 minutes for preparation. Baking requires around 10 minutes per batch. You can make up to 5 dozen oatmeal cookies with the following ingredients.

- Hot water; 2 tablespoons

- Ground flaxseed; 1 tablespoon

- Dried chopped plums; 1 cup

- Dates (chopped); 1 cup

- Raisins; Half cup

- Softened butter; 1/3 cup

- Brown sugar; ¾ cup

- Large egg

- Vanilla extract; 2 teaspoons

- Applesauce (unsweetened); Half cup

- Maple syrup; ¼ cup

- Orange zest; 1 tablespoon

- Oats (quick-cooking); 3 cups

- All-purpose flour; 1 cup

- Whole-wheat flour; Half cup

- Baking soda; 1 teaspoon

- Ground cinnamon; 1 teaspoon

- Salt; Half teaspoon

- Ground nutmeg; ¼ teaspoon

- Ground cloves; ¼ teaspoon

Combine water and the flaxseed in a bowl. Combine the raisins, dates, and plums into another bowl. Cover with hot water. Let mixtures of flaxseed and plum stand for 10 minutes.

Then, mix butter and brown sugar in a bowl until it gets fluffy. Beat in Vanilla and Egg. Beat in applesauce, orange zest, and maple syrup. Combine the oats, flours, baking soda, salt, cinnamon, butter, cloves, and nutmeg; slowly apply and blend well to the creamed mixture. Drain the mixture of the plum; add the mixture of the plum and the flaxseed to the flour.

Drop by teaspoonfuls 2 inches apart on a lightly greased baking sheet. Bake it at 350° for about 8 to 11 minutes. Let it cool for 2 minutes before you remove it from pans to the wire racks.

31. Peanut Butter Cake

The preparation time for this cake is 20 minutes. Baking requires 15 minutes along with cooling.

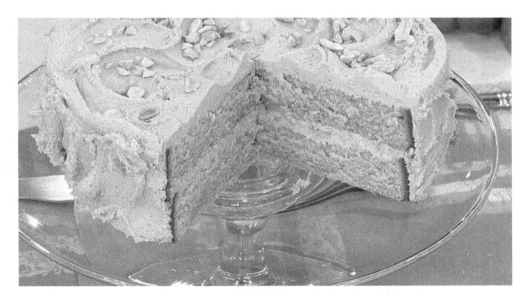

- Cubed butter; 6 tablespoons

- Peanut butter (creamy); Half cup

- Water; 1 cup

- All-purpose flour; 2 cups

- Sugar; 1 ½ cups

- Buttermilk; Half cup

- Applesauce (unsweetened); ¼ cup

- Large eggs (2); slightly beaten

- Baking powder; 1 ¼ teaspoon

- Vanilla extract; 1 teaspoon

- Salt; Half teaspoon

- Baking soda; ¼ teaspoon

For the cake's frosting, you need the following ingredients.

- Cubed butter; ¼ cup

- Peanut butter (creamy); ¼ cup

- Milk (fat-free); 2 tablespoons

- Confectioner sugar; 1 ¾ cup

- Vanilla extract; 1 teaspoon

Mix butter, water, and peanut butter in a saucepan and bring it to a boil. Remove it from heat immediately. Add flour, applesauce, sugar, eggs, buttermilk, salt, vanilla, baking soda, and baking powder. Mix it well.

Pour the mixture into a 15 by 10 by 1-inch baking pan covered with cooking spray. Bake it at 375° for about 15 to 20 minutes or wait until it is golden brown. Cool it for 20 to 30 minutes on a wire rack.

In a saucepan, mix peanut butter and butter on medium heat and then add milk. Boil it and then remove it from heat. Slowly add in vanilla and confectioner sugar and mix it well until it gets smooth. Spread it over a warm cake. Allow it to cool and then you can refrigerate the leftovers.

You can add nuts too!

32. Zucchini Bread – Diabetic

This bread is good and healthy for diabetes patients. It is low in sugar and low in carbs. And it is going to keep you healthy as well.

You need:

- Egg white; ¾ cup

- Applesauce (unsweetened); Half cup

- Melted butter (fat-free); Half cup

- Shredded Zucchini; 2 cups

- Shredded Carrot; Half cup

- Brown sugar; 6 tablespoons

- Baking powder; 1 teaspoon

- Baking soda; 1 teaspoon

- Cinnamon; 1 teaspoon

- Nutmeg; 1 teaspoon

- Salt; Half teaspoon

- Vanilla extract; 2 teaspoons

- Chopped walnuts; ¼ cup

- Whole-wheat flour; 2 cups

Preheat the oven to 350 degrees.

Then, grease and then flour two medium pans for loaves.

In a bowl combine brown sugar, egg, sugar, margarine, and apple sauce.

Then, add baking powder, cinnamon, baking soda, salt, nutmeg, and vanilla.

Then, add flour slowly and add shredded zucchini, nuts, and carrots.

Use a mixer or your hands to beat the mixture and pour the mixture into the loaf pans.

Bake it for 45 minutes. After that, let it cool.

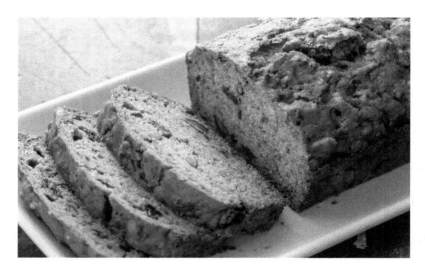

33. Berry Parfait

The perfect period for this parfait is mid-summer, as the northern forests are dense with blueberries. The total time required for this parfait is around 15 to 20 minutes which includes preparation as well.

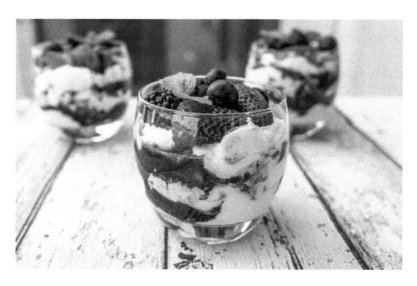

- Fresh strawberries; 2 cups; cut in half

- Fresh blueberries; 2 cups

- Walnut raspberry vinaigrette; 4 teaspoons

- Greek yogurt (strawberry or vanilla) fat-free; ¾ cup

- Fresh mint (minced); 2 teaspoons

- Shredded coconut (unsweetened); Optional

Put the blueberries and strawberries in separate cups. Drizzle Vinaigrette (2 teaspoons) on both the berries. Blend mint and yogurt in a bowl.

Place strawberries into four cups for the parfait. Cover each with blueberries and yogurt mixture. You can top it with shredded coconut as well if you want to!

34. Cinnamon Bars

In this recipe, the Classic bar follows good-for-you ingredients. If you can then keep them in a tin for a day after the bars are prepared. The next day, I think they taste much better. You can easily make around 2 dozen bars using the following ingredients. However, the total time required for the ingredient preparation is 20 to 25 minutes and 15 to 20 minutes for baking along with cooling.

- Whole wheat flour; Half cup

- All-purpose flour; Half cup

- Sugar; Half cup

- Ground cinnamon; 1 ½ teaspoon

- Baking powder; 1 ¼ teaspoon

- Baking soda; ¼ teaspoon

- Large egg; beaten

- Canola oil; 1/3 cup

- Applesauce (unsweetened); ¼ cup

- Honey; ¼ cup

- Walnuts (chopped); 1 cup

  Now, for the icing, you need the following ingredients.

- Melted butter; 2 tablespoons

- Water; 1 tablespoon

- Honey; 2 tablespoons

- Vanilla extract; 1 teaspoon

- Confectioner sugar; 1 cup

Preheat the oven to 350°. In a bowl, mix flours, baking powder, sugar, baking soda, and cinnamon. Mix oil, egg, honey, and applesauce in a bowl. Put it into the dry ingredients as it gets creamy and then add in walnuts.

Spread the batter into a 13 by 9 inches baking pan greased with cooking spray. Bake for about 15 to 20 minutes. You will know when it is done!

Now, combine your icing ingredients and spread it over the warm bars. Let the bars cool down entirely before you cut them!

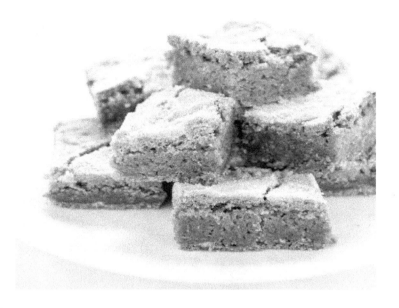

35. Banana Bread

It is a good snack for people with diabetes or prediabetic persons. Preparation time is about 10 to 15 minutes and baking requires almost 1 hour.

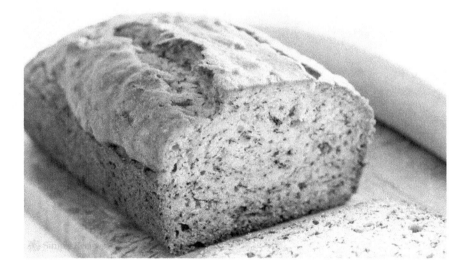

- Bananas (large); 2

- 2 Eggs

- Rapeseed oil; 4 tablespoons

- Vanilla extract; 1 teaspoon

- Brown sugar; 100 grams

- Flour (whole meal); 150 grams

- Baking powder; 2 teaspoons

- Mixed spice; 1 teaspoon (heaped)

- Walnuts (chopped); 50 grams

Preheat your oven to 170°C. Mash your bananas and once done, add eggs and then mix it well. Then add the vanilla extract, sugar, and oil. Mix it well.

Add in the flour, mixed spice, and baking powder and then add the chopped walnuts.

Pour the batter into a 2 pounds loaf tin, place the nuts on the top of the loaf, and bake it for 50 to 55 minutes, until a toothpick inserted into its center comes out neat.

Let it cool for 10 minutes in the pan and then you can remove it for it to cool down completely.

Tips:

You can also add other spices to it such as ground cinnamon or ground ginger, or you can use almonds instead of walnuts.

Freezing tips: You can freeze its slices in foil once it is prepared!

36.Chunky Apple Cake

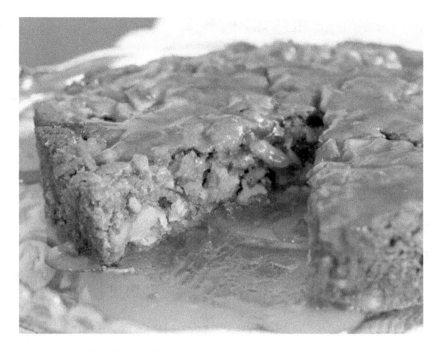

The preparation time for the ingredients required for this cake is approx. 30 minutes and 20 to 25 minutes for baking along with cooling. You can make 20 servings with the following ingredients.

- Large eggs; 2

- Brown sugar; Half cup

- Melted butter; 6 tablespoons

- Sugar; ¼ cup

- Vanilla extract; 2 teaspoons

- All-purpose flour; 2 cups

- Ground cinnamon; 2 teaspoons

- Baking powder; 1 teaspoon

- Baking soda; 1 teaspoon

- Salt; ¼ teaspoon

- Apples (shredded); 4; medium-sized

- Pecans (chopped); ¾ cup

Preheat your oven to 350 ° C. Coat a baking pan with cooking spray, 13 by 9 inches. Beat eggs, brown sugar, melted butter, sugar, and vanilla in a large bowl, until well mixed. Whisk sugar, flour, baking soda, salt, and baking powder in another bowl; slowly beat into a mixture of eggs. Stir in pecans and apples.

Switch to a prepared pan. Bake for 25-30 minutes or until the inserted toothpick in the center comes out of the cake clean. Cool on a wire rack, in the pan.

37. Elephant Ear Cookies

Now, this is something even your children will love to eat as a snack.

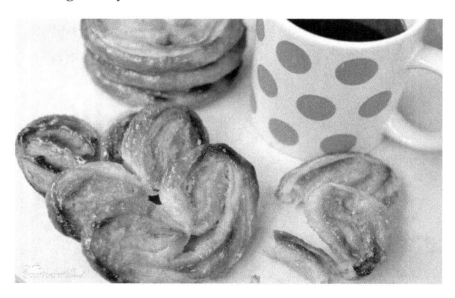

You need 35 to 40 minutes for the preparation and 10 to 15 minutes for baking these marvelous cookies. You can make approx. 2 dozen biscuits with the following ingredients.

- Active yeast (dry); ¼ oz.

- Warm water; ¼ cup

- All-purpose flour; 2 cups

- Sugar; 4 and a half teaspoons

- Salt; Half teaspoon

- Cubed butter (cold); 1/3 cup

- Milk (fat-free or low-fat); 1/3 cup

- Egg yolk (large egg)

For the filling, you need the following ingredients.

- Softened butter; 2 tablespoons

- Sugar; Half cup

- Ground cinnamon; 2 teaspoons

How to make cinnamon sugar? Here are the ingredients that you need to mix!

- Ground cinnamon; ¾ teaspoon

- Sugar; Half cup

Dissolve yeast in a ¼ cup warm. Mix the flour, salt, and sugar in a bowl; break into butter until you can see the crumbly texture. Stir in the yeast mixture the egg yolk and milk; add to the flour mixture, stir it to form the dough (your dough is going to be sticky). Cover it with plastic wrap. Then, cool down for 2 hours approx.

Preheat the oven until 375 ° C. Turn the dough on a floured wooden mat; roll the dough into a rectangle of 18 by 10 inches. Layer to about 1/4 inches with melted butter. For rims. Mix cinnamon and sugar; scatter on milk. Roll up type jelly-roll, starting with its long side; pinch the seam to close. Cut into 24 parts, crosswise. Cover slices with plastic wrap up to flattening level.

In a bowl, mix the cinnamon sugar ingredients. Place a strip of waxed paper 6 inches square on a working surface; sprinkle it with cinnamon sugar. Then, top it with one piece of dough; add cinnamon sugar (half teaspoon) to sprinkle on the dough. Roll the dough down to a diameter of 4 inches. Flip the dough onto a baking sheet lined with the cooking spray using waxed paper. Repeat the steps with the remaining ingredients, separating the slices by 2 inches. Bake for 7 to 9 minutes or to brown until golden. Cool on rack wire.

38.Masala Bread Rolls – Whole Wheat

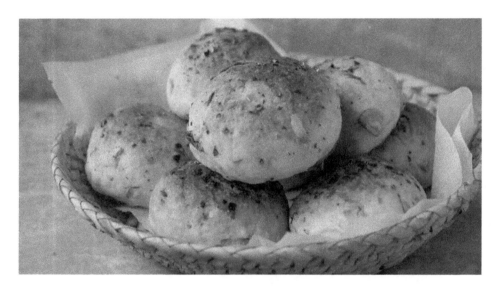

For these delicious bread rolls, different steps require different time. Preparation is done in approx. 10 to 15 minutes. Cooking requires about 2 to 5 minutes and 25 to 35 minutes for baking. You can make Nine bread rolls using the following ingredients.

- Whole wheat flour; 2 cups

- Instant yeast; 2 teaspoons

- Sugar; Half teaspoon

- Butter (low-fat); 2 teaspoons

- Salt for taste

- Melted butter (low fat) for brushing; ¼ teaspoon

To prepare the masala for the bread rolls, you need the following ingredients.

- Oil; 1 teaspoon

- Onions (chopped); ¼ cup

- Garlic (chopped); 1 tablespoon

- Green chilies (chopped); a Half tablespoon

- Chopped cilantro; ½ cup

- Turmeric powder; ¼ teaspoon

- Salt for taste

To prepare the masala:

Heat the oil or low-fat butter in a pan. If it is a non-stick pan, then it is better. Then, add onions, green chilies, and garlic in the pan. Cook it for 1 minute on medium flame.

Then, add cilantro, turmeric, salt, and chili powder. Mix it properly. Then cook it for 1 minute on a medium flame.

Put it aside to cool it down and your masala is ready.

To prepare the Bread Rolls:

In a shallow pot, mix the yeast with warm water, cover it with a lid and leave it aside for ten minutes. Now, in a deep tub, add the whole wheat flour, salt, butter, and the yeast mixture and knead it into a gentle dough with warm water.

Cover with a moist muslin cloth over the dough and held aside for 20 minutes or until the dough rises a bit.

Now apply the masala powdered, and knead properly.

Divide the dough into 9 equal parts and roll each part into a disk, then put the dough on the grated baking tray.

Then, over them with a moist cloth of muslin and keep them in a warm spot for around 30 minutes or until they grow up.

Bake them in a preheated oven for 20 to 25 minutes, at 200 degrees. Brush the melted butter to the bread rolls and serve them!

39. Oatmeal Bread – Gingerbread

The preparation time for this bread is 10 minutes and approx. 3 hours for baking! You can easily make 1 loaf using the following ingredients.

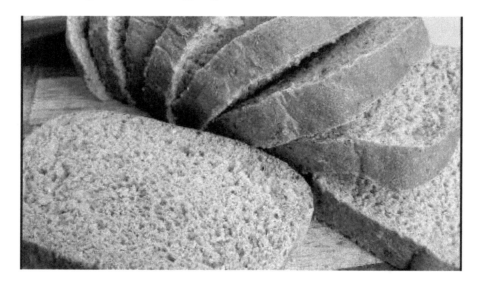

- Water; 1 cup + 1 tablespoon

- Molasses; Half cup

- Canola oil; 1 tablespoon

- Bread flour; 3 cups

- Oats; 1 cup

- Ground cinnamon; 1 and a half teaspoon

- Ground ginger; 1 teaspoon or Half more

- Salt; 1 teaspoon

- Orange zest (grated); Half teaspoon

- Ground nutmeg; ¼ teaspoon

- Ground cloves; ¼ teaspoon

- Active yeast; ¼ oz.

Layer all ingredients in the bread machine pan in the order suggested by the maker. Pick a simple environment for the bread. Pick the color of the crust and size of the loaf, if appropriate.

Bake according to the instructions of the bread machine (check the dough after five minutes of mixing; apply 1 to 2 spoons of water or flour if necessary).

40.Light Chocolate Pudding

This pudding is creamy and it is light just as promised! You need 10 minutes for preparation and 15 to 20 minutes for cooking it along with cooling. You can make 4 servings out of the following ingredients.

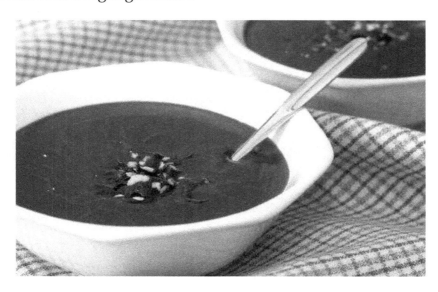

- Cornstarch; 3 tablespoons

- Sugar; 2 tablespoons

- Baking cocoa; 2 tablespoons

- Salt; 1/8 teaspoon

- Soy milk (chocolate); 2 cups

- Vanilla extract; 1 teaspoon

Add the cornstarch, cocoa, sugar, salt in a hot, heavy saucepan. Whisk in some milk. Cook and mix over medium heat until bubbly and thickened. Reduce heat to low; boil and stir for 2 minutes.

Remove the saucepan from heat and then stir vanilla in. Cool for 15 minutes.

Transfer to plates for dessert. Cover, refrigerate, for 30 minutes, or until cold.

41. Lemon Cheese Bars

These delicious bars take 15 to 20 minutes for preparation along with 25 to 30 minutes for baking and more time for cooling. You can prepare 2 dozen bars with the following ingredients.

- Lemon cake mix; 1 packet

- Egg substitute; Half cup

- Canola oil; 1/3 cup

- Cream cheese (low-fat); 8 oz.

- Sugar; 1/3 cup

- Lemon juice; 1 teaspoon

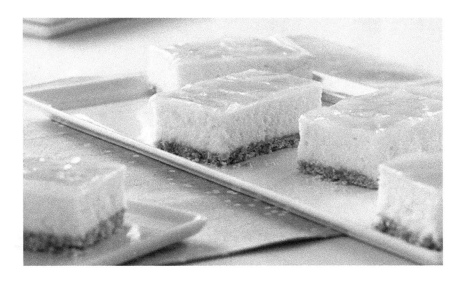

Preheat your oven to 350 ° C. Combine cake mix, the egg substitute, and oil in a deep bowl; combine until smooth. To top off-reserve 1/2 cup mixture. Place the excess mixture into the bottom of a baking sheet with cooking spray lined with 13 by 9 inches. Bake for 11-13 minutes or until light brown around the bottom.

Mix cream cheese, sugar, and lemon juice in a medium cup, until smooth. Add the remaining egg substitute; beat only until blended at a low level. Disseminate over salt. Crumble is reserved for filling over top.

Bake for 11-13 minutes, or until it is ready to complete. Cooldown 1 hour on a wire rack. Split these into plates. Keep the leftover in your refrigerator.

42. Almond Hazelnut Biscotti

You need 30 minutes for preparation and 30 minutes for baking. You can make approx. 2 dozen biscotti using the following ingredients.

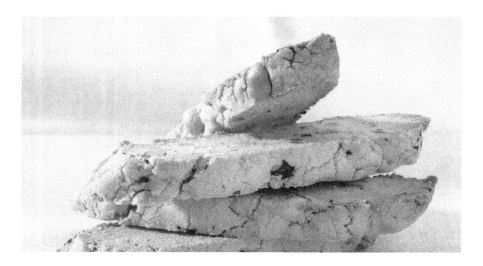

- Large eggs; 2

- Sugar; ¾ cup

- Vanilla extract; 2 teaspoons

- Almond extract; ¾ teaspoon

- All-purpose flour; 1 2/3 cup

- Salt; ¼ teaspoon

- Baking soda; Half teaspoon

- Hazelnuts (chopped and toasted); 2/3 cup

- Almonds (sliced and toasted); ¼ cup

Toast almonds, bake for 5-10 minutes in a shallow pan in a 350 ° oven, or roast over low heat in a skillet until well browned and stirring regularly.

Preheat your oven to 350 ° C. Beat eggs, sugar, and spices in a bowl, until well combined. Whisk the rice, baking soda and salt together in another bowl; slowly whisk in the egg mixture. Stir in the nuts (the mixture becomes stiff).

Divide the batter into two. Using lightly floured palms, form each section on a parchment-lined baking sheet into a rectangle measuring 9 by 2 inches. Bake for about 20 minutes, until golden brown.

Cool on wire racks till firm on pans. Reduce the level on the oven to 325 °. Move rectangles boiled to a cutting plate. Cut diagonally through 3/4-in, use a serrated knife. Sliced slices. Put them on baking sheets, cut the side down.

Bake for 5-7 minutes per leg, until lightly browned. Remove to wire racks from the pans; cool down completely. Store in a container that is airtight.

43. Banana Cereal Popsicles

15 minutes for preparation and almost 1 hour for freezing. Make 8 pops with the following ingredients.

- Strawberry yogurt; ¾ cup

- Bananas (medium-sized) cut in half; 4

- Cereal; Fruity Pebbles; 2 cups

- Wooden sticks; 8

Put yogurt and cereal in individual, shallow bowls. Attach pop sticks to the banana from the side that you cut. Dip the bananas in yogurt, then roll them to cover in cereal. Switch to waxed baking sheets lined with parchment.

Freeze up for around 1 hour, before solid. Transfer to containers with airtight freezer; seal containers, and return pops to the freezer.

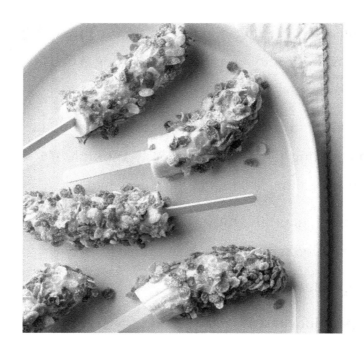

Tips:

• Switch it to vanilla yogurt or Cocoa Pebbles.

• This basic formula accounts for the use of mature and sweet but yet strong bananas. Search for bananas with little to no green, with no gray or black stains on them. This is a clever way of utilizing a load of extra bananas.

Conclusion

A low-carb diet can help diabetics control their blood sugar rates easier. Carbohydrates are more likely to boost blood glucose than other products, suggesting the body will generate more insulin to absorb them. Reducing the intake of carb may help to stabilize blood glucose. It can also counteract some of the other diabetes effects, such as heart diseases or weight gain. More than that, low-carb diets often bear other hazards of deficits in vitamins and minerals. Low carb diets are difficult for certain people to adhere to overtime. People should try to speak to a doctor before making major dietary adjustments, especially those that involve diabetes control.

While the link among sugar and diabetes remains uncertain, a reduction in the diet's added sugar and refined food may help an individual avoid type 2 diabetes. Other adjustments to the lifestyle can help decrease the risk of type 2 diabetes or assist people with diabetes to deal with their problems and avoid complications.

A low-carb diet may help diabetes sufferers prevent complications. This will help maintain the blood pressure down, rising energy slumps, support weight reduction, and even change the disease path. A low-carb diet can be the first line of therapy for patients who choose to delay drugs, or whose doctor has just newly identified diabetes. Low-carb diets are not an unhealthy low-carb diet for everyone — like living off fried, fatty meats — might be even more harmful to a person's health than lots of carbs.

Similarly, a person must be able to stick to a long-term low-carb diet to fully reap its benefits. Please speak to a specialist or dietitian before carrying out some new diet. People may consider keeping a list of their symptoms and what they've consumed, to assess how the diet affects their long-time wellbeing.

CPSIA information can be obtained
at www.ICGtesting.com
Printed in the USA
LVHW110717230122
709139LV00013B/874